SWISS BALL
CORE TRAINING

PumpOne

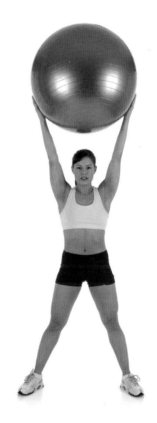

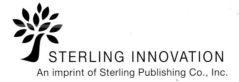

STERLING INNOVATION
An imprint of Sterling Publishing Co., Inc.

New York / London
www.sterlingpublishing.com

PumpOne

STERLING and the distinctive Sterling logo are registered trademarks of Sterling Publishing Co., Inc.

10 9 8 7 6 5 4 3 2 1

Published by Sterling Publishing Co., Inc.
387 Park Avenue South, New York, NY 10016

© 2007 by PumpOne

Distributed in Canada by Sterling Publishing
c/o Canadian Manda Group, 165 Dufferin Street
Toronto, Ontario, Canada M6K 3H6
Distributed in the United Kingdom by GMC Distribution Services
Castle Place, 166 High Street, Lewes, East Sussex, England BN7 1XU
Distributed in Australia by Capricorn Link (Australia) Pty. Ltd.
P.O. Box 704, Windsor, NSW 2756, Australia

Modeling by Dilia Jelen and Mike Nicholioson
Photographs by Craig Schlossberg/PumpOne
Text by Declan Condron

PumpOne

Design by Beth Nori

Printed in China
All rights reserved

Sterling ISBN-13: 978-1-4027-4949-0
         ISBN-10: 1-4027-4949-X

The exercise programs described in this book are based on well-established practices proven to be effective for over-all health and fitness, but they are not a substitute for personalized advice from a qualified practitioner. Always consult with a qualified health care professional in matters relating to your health before beginning this or any exercise program. This is especially important if you are pregnant or nursing, if you are elderly, or if you have any chronic or recurring medical condition. As with any exercise program, if at any point during your workout you begin to feel faint, dizzy, or have physical discomfort, you should stop immediately and consult a physician.

The purpose of this book is to educate and is sold with the understanding that the author and the publisher shall have neither liability nor responsibility for any injury caused or alleged to be caused directly or indirectly by the information contained in this book.

For information about custom editions, special sales, premium and corporate purchases, please contact Sterling Special Sales Department at 800-805-5489 or specialsales@sterlingpub.com.

CONTENTS

Introduction 4

The Core Defined 5

Safety Precautions 6

Equipment 8

How This Book Works 8

Getting Started 10

Warming Up and Cooling Down . 12

Workout 1 13

Workout 2 23

Workout 3 33

Workout 4 43

Stretching 53

Index 63

INTRODUCTION

Welcome to the *Swiss Ball Core Training* book. This book is designed to provide multiple workouts that are performed using only a Swiss ball and one's body weight. These workouts can be done anywhere: at home, while traveling, or at the gym (most gyms will have Swiss balls in different sizes).

Using a Swiss ball for exercising is not a new concept. The ball has been used for rehabilitation and physical therapy for many years. It was first introduced in Switzerland in 1963, earning the name Swiss ball. (It's sometimes called a gymnastic ball, or a fit ball.) Swiss balls gained popularity in gyms and health clubs in the 1990s and are now standard equipment in most exercise facilities.

This book on Swiss ball training is not just a list of exercises but it provides specific, graduated, progressive workouts. It will guide you on the proper form for each exercise as it takes you through each workout.

So What's the Big Deal with the Ball?

Why use a Swiss ball? It looks slippery and unstable. Might be a little dangerous? What can it do for you? Swiss balls are completely safe and offer many benefits for fitness training. Actually, it's the very instability of a Swiss ball that makes it such an excellent exercise tool. Just by sitting on the ball, you activate the stabilizer muscles of your core.

Some Benefits:

Increased Neuromuscular Functioning

The neuromuscular system is the connection between the brain, central nervous system, and the muscles. To perform a movement or action your brain sends a message via the nervous system to the muscles to go into action. Using a Swiss ball involves greater muscle activity and ignites more and better-quality messages moving through the nerve-muscle conduit from the brain.

Improvements in coordination and proprioception

As the brain communicates with the muscles, the muscles talk back to the brain. This is called proprioception, and sometimes kinesthesia. Muscles sense where your limbs are in space and signal to your brain: "your left arm is above your head," or "your right leg is straight out in front." A Swiss ball challenges proprioception because it is less stable than a bench and requires quick adjustment to maintain balance. This messaging between the brain and muscles builds better coordination and proprioception.

Develop better muscle synergy

Contrary to popular belief, a muscle group does not work by itself. Muscle groups work together to facilitate movement, and also to stabilize and support inert body parts. For example, during a biceps curl, your biceps muscles contract to move your arm, while your deltoid muscles help the movement and also stabilize your shoulders. Meanwhile, the triceps work to control the speed of the movement. Using a Swiss ball can help develop better synergy between muscle groups.

Variety

Our bodies are very smart machines. When our brain asks us to move, our brain figures out the easiest way to do it. Asked to perform a movement again and again, it becomes increasingly easy. Changing the task slightly gives our bodies a new challenge: to figure out a better way to meet new requirements. A Swiss ball is a great tool for changing a workout and giving the body new stimuli.

THE CORE DEFINED

Our body's core is defined as the deep abdominal and spinal muscles that support the spine and help to maintain a neutral position during movement. This is just partly true. The definition of the core can be expanded to include almost all the muscles of the torso. This includes the smaller deep muscles, such as the *transverse abdominus* and *multifidius*, but also the larger muscles such as the *rectus abdominus, quadratus lumborum* (lower back muscles that maintain spinal and pelvic balance), internal and external *obliques*, the *erector spinae*, the *latissimus dorsi*, and *ilio-psoas* muscles.

This muscular core acts like a corset that can stabilize, move, resist movement, and lend support all at once. Remember, muscle groups don't act in isolation; they act in synergy to produce the best movement strategy possible. Therefore, core muscles work together to produce the most efficient movement, but not always the safest movement.

The Swiss ball and the back

Back pain is one of the most common physical problems in the United States today. It is estimated that eight out of ten people will suffer some form of back pain at some stage in their life. These statistics are not very encouraging, but there is hope: With a good overall fitness lifestyle, we can greatly reduce this risk. Originally the Swiss ball was used to rehabilitate adults with orthopedic injuries, including back injuries. Any of us can go a long way in keeping our backs strong, healthy, and free of injury by using a Swiss ball to strengthen core muscle groups, increase their neuromuscular functioning, improve their proprioception and coordination, and develop overall synergy.

A Word about posture

Posture can be defined as the position or bearing of the body. It refers to the overall alignment of body parts to each other when standing in a relaxed position. Posture is the result of many processes and tensions in the body. It becomes a measure of overall balance. With good posture a person's overall structure is in good mechanical balance. Bad posture results when some areas of the body don't permit the appropriate mechanical ability. Poor posture can lead to mechanical problems, dysfunctions, and pain.

Let's take a look at the spine. If a person can position his spine so his vertebrae are aligned over one another without lateral curvature, and his muscles, ligaments, and tendons balance his weight with minimal effort, he is in a good neutral spinal posture with respect to the force of gravity. If, however, one vertebra is off track, or one muscle is not functioning, alignment is off, which can cause excessive stress on the spine, resulting in injury.

Exercise, stretching, massage, and careful training can help to restore balance and good posture. A Swiss ball is an excellent training stimulus. In these workouts, you will see the phrase "maintain a neutral spine." This refers to having good posture throughout the spine, having everything aligned naturally with all the soft tissues—muscles, tendons, ligaments, and nerves—remaining strong.

SAFETY PRECAUTIONS

As with any exercise program, safety is of the utmost importance. The last thing you want to do is to injure yourself trying to get into better shape and improve your health. Before you start we recommend you do the following:

Talk to your doctor

Always consult your doctor before starting a fitness program, especially if you have or have had a chronic medical condition, are taking any medications, or are pregnant.

Immediately stop exercising if you feel pain, faintness, dizziness, or shortness of breath. Wait awhile. You may decide to quit for the day, or resume slowly.

Get equipped

Check the condition of the Swiss ball and make sure you choose the right ball for your body size. Follow the manufacturer's instructions for inflation.

Read all warnings and instructions on the proper use and maintenance of the ball before you begin.

Make room

Make sure you have enough space to exercise, and avoid exercising on slippery surfaces. Be aware of the surrounding areas, other people, and any obstacles that might cause a fall.

Suit up

Wear appropriate exercise clothing that is neither too baggy nor too tight. Also be sure to wear some form of footwear. Sneakers are comfortable and have a nonslip sole.

Warm-up and cool down

Always warm-up for at least five minutes before starting any workout. Warming up gets the body ready to exercise and increases its core temperature and muscle elasticity. A warm-up can consist of some light cardiovascular work such as jogging on a treadmill and/or a few light sets of an exercise before you start the workout sets. Also be sure to cool down and stretch after your workout. This will help relax your muscles and return them to their resting length, and reduce to normal your core temperature. We have included a number of specific stretches to choose from after your workouts.

Have water on hand

It's a good idea to eat something at least two hours before exercising, and always to have water on hand while you are working out. Right after working out is a great time to replenish the body's energy supplies, while you relax and rest.

EQUIPMENT

The only equipment needed for the workouts in this book is a Swiss Ball and your own body weight.

Swiss balls come in various sizes and colors. Be sure to choose the correct ball for you. Manufacturers provide size guidelines based on height. A general rule of thumb is that when seated on the ball, your hips should be slightly higher than your knees, and your feet should be flat on the floor. The ball provided in this kit is 55 cm.

The following size chart can be used as a general rule:

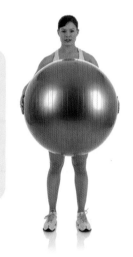

BALL SIZE GUIDELINES FOR EXERCISE	
Height	Ball Size
Under 5'2" (1.57 m)	45 cm
5'3"–5'8" (1.60 m–1.72 m)	55 cm
5'9"–6'2" (1.75 m–1.88 m)	65 cm
Above 6'3" (1.90 m)	75 cm

Inflate the ball according to the manufacturers' guidelines. Most balls come with a hand or foot pump.

HOW THIS BOOK WORKS

This book is organized as a progressive exercise plan. Like a personal trainer, it is a guide to what exercises to perform, in which order, and when to advance to a new workout to keep you working toward a stronger, fitter body.

The book contains four separate workouts with ten different exercises in each. These workouts can be performed at different intensities by varying the number of repetitions and sets and the amount of rest between sets. The book offers two different intensity levels for each workout: the **Express track** and the **Intense track**. The **Express track** uses **two sets of fifteen reps per exercise**, and should take approximately **twenty minutes to complete** a workout. The **Intense track** uses **three**

sets of twenty reps per exercise, and should take approximately **forty minutes to complete** a workout. Both tracks are designed to help you lose weight while increasing muscle strength and definition.

The four workouts provide an overall exercise plan, which becomes more difficult as you get fitter. We suggest performing two to three workout sessions per week. Begin alternating workouts one and two for the first two weeks and work your way up to workouts three and four. Just as the body needs variety, it also needs consistency. Perform each workout a few times. Workouts three and four are more challenging and may take some time to master, so take your time and enjoy the journey.

There are ten stretching exercises at the end of the workouts. They can be performed all together as a separate stretching workout. Or, you can choose three or four of these stretches to perform as part of your cooldown after each workout.

Accompanying this book is a DVD that contains the same exercise and stretching workouts. You can use the DVD to view the workouts on your television and perform the exercises in the comfort of your own home. There is also an installation program on the DVD that will allow you to add these workouts to your computer and sync them to your image-ready handheld device such as an iPod, iPod nano, or Treo. This allows you to take your workouts with you wherever you go in an easy portable format.

A plan for total health

Before you reach for your Swiss ball, take a few minutes to consider the whole picture. Exercising with a Swiss ball should be part of an overall plan for total health, a plan that takes some dedication and hard work. No one gets fit and strong overnight. Using a Swiss ball is a great tool for achieving strength and fitness, but it is not a cure-all. An overall health plan should incorporate a number of practices and habits that have an impact on your body. There are five essential components to a health plan—strength training; cardiovascular training; flexibility and mobility; a healthy nutrition plan; and adequate rest and recovery. An effective exercise program depends on all five of these measures. The right emphasis on each depends on your individual goals.

For more digital training programs in all areas of fitness visit **www.PumpOne.com.** You can choose from different fitness goals and levels to find other exercise programs to complement the Swiss Ball Core Training program.

GETTING STARTED

Ready to get started? You have your equipment and are eager to perform those first repetitions. Consider a few last tips before you begin. If this is your first time using a Swiss ball or if it's been a while, take some time to get familiar with sitting and lying and eventually kneeling on it. Take it easy at first. Practice these three positions:

1. Sit on the ball.

Sit on the top center of the ball with your feet flat on the floor. Your hips should be slightly higher than your knees. Keep your head up and look straight ahead, aligning your shoulders over your hips. Be conscious of the position of your spine at all times. Do not let your shoulders roll forward or flex your lower back. This will help you establish good posture along your spine while seated on the ball.

2. Lie on the ball.

Lie facedown with the ball under your midsection and your hands and feet on the floor. Practice rolling forward and backward, lifting your hands or feet as you roll. When you feel comfortable with these movements, move side to side, and work up to lying on the ball without your hands or feet touching the floor.

Next, turn over on your back and center the ball between your shoulder blades. Place your feet flat on the floor and your hands on your hips. Keep your hips level with your shoulders. This requires you to contract your abdominal and core muscles and will be used a lot in the exercises.

3. Kneel on the ball.

For this position, keep something sturdy like a chair or bench close by to help with balance. Place both hands and one knee on top of the ball. Slowly lift your other leg off the floor, and place your other knee on the ball. You should now be on all fours atop the ball. Now place one hand on the chair to help stabilize yourself, and lift the other hand off the ball. Move your upper body upright. Just as in the seated position, you should be conscious of the position of your spine. Do not let your shoulders roll forward or flex your lower back. Take your hand off the support and practice holding your body upright. You will move around some, so try to relax and find your center of balance.

Once you are comfortable with these positions on the ball, you are ready to start working out. Be sure to concentrate on your breathing as you perform the exercises. Whether you breathe in or out as you lift the ball is not as important as remembering to breathe. Do not hold your breath.

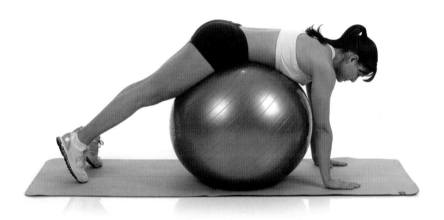

WARMING UP AND COOLING DOWN

A warm-up is a crucial part of any exercise program. The importance of a structured warm-up cannot be overstated. It is essential for getting the body ready for activity and helping prevent injury. Warming up before working out prepares you for strenuous activity by increasing the temperature of both the body's core and muscles. Increasing muscle temperature helps to loosen the muscles, making them more supple and flexible.

Warming up also increases your heart rate and the rate of blood flow to your muscles, increasing the delivery of oxygen and nutrients to your muscles and helping prepare them and other tissues for activity.

A concise warm-up should last 10 to 15 minutes. It should target all areas of the body, starting with gentle activity such as light cardiovascular work. It should gradually increase in intensity, building up to movements similar to the exercises in the workout. Static stretching before working out is optional.

Just as important as warming up before exercising is a good cooldown afterward. Cooling down helps return your core temperature to normal and helps muscles relax and return to their original length. Stretching during a cooldown can help to increase muscle and joint range of motion, which will improve flexibility and may reduce muscle soreness. There are a number of specific stretches at the end of the workouts that target the major muscle groups that have been used. Choose three or four stretches to perform at the end of each workout.

Exercise 1
OVERHEAD SQUAT

1 Start in a squat position with your feet flat and your back in a neutral position. Hold the ball out in front of you at waist height.

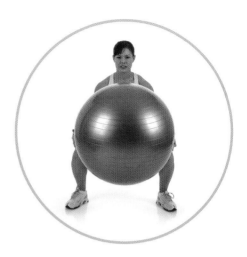

2 Stand tall and raise the ball overhead, extending your arms fully.

Be sure to squat as low as you can and stretch as high as you can.

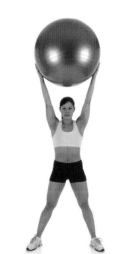

Hints

Keep your head up and look straight ahead throughout the movement. Do not look down at the floor or your feet.

Make sure to keep your feet flat on the floor with your heels down as you move up and down.

Exercise 2
WALL PUSH-UP

1 Stand with your feet hip-width apart, facing a wall, holding the ball against the wall at chest height. Position your hands on the ball with your elbows bent and your chest nearly touching the ball.

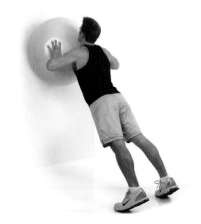

2 Push your body up and away from the ball until your arms are fully extended.

Slowly lower your body back to the starting position.

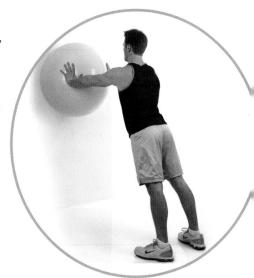

Hints
Keep your back straight by contracting your core muscles. Do not round your lower back.

Move all the way up and all the way down, until your chest is nearly touching the ball.

Exercise 3
BALL CRUNCH

1 Lie with your mid-back on the ball. Keep your head and neck off the ball and your feet flat on the floor.

Place your hands at the sides of your head.

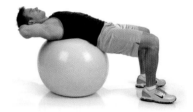

2 Lift your head and shoulders up and away from the ball, contracting your abdominals.

Roll your upper body back over the ball, returning to the starting position.

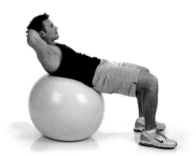

Hints

Make an effort to control the movement through your midsection, and avoid jerky movements.

Don't use your hands to pull up your head and neck.

Raise only your head and shoulders, not your whole back.

Exercise 4
LUNGE

1 Stand upright with your arms extended, holding the ball overhead.

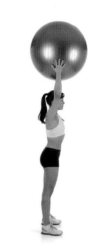

2 Step forward and drop your back knee toward the floor, bending at the hip and knee.

Lean slightly forward, keeping all your weight on the front foot, still holding the ball overhead.

Push off with the front foot to return to the starting position, and repeat with your other leg.

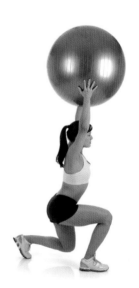

Hints

The position of your back is very important in squatting exercises. Always maintain a neutral position, neither rounding your lower back nor overarching it.

Keep your head up looking straight ahead with your shoulders back. This will help prevent rounding the upper back. Place your weight over the leg you step onto and push off this leg to return to the central position.

Exercise 5
ROLL OUT

1 Kneel on the mat with your forearms on the ball, your elbows bent, and your chest nearly touching the ball.

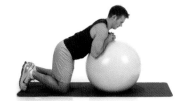

2 Push the ball forward, extending your arms and keeping your upper body rigid.

Pull the ball back, drawing your elbows in until you reach the starting position.

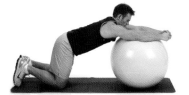

Hints

Maintain a neutral spine by looking down and not moving your head.

Control the movement through your midsection, and avoid jerky movements. This requires you to keep your abdominal and core muscles contracted throughout the exercise.

Exercise 6
KNEELING OBLIQUE CRUNCH

1 Lie on one side on the ball with one knee on the mat and the other leg stretched out to the side.

Place your hands at the sides of your head.

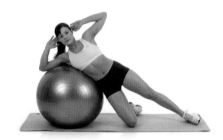

2 Raise your upper body up and off the ball, bringing your outside elbow down to your side.

Lower your body, returning to the starting position. Lie over the ball. Complete your reps and repeat on the other side.

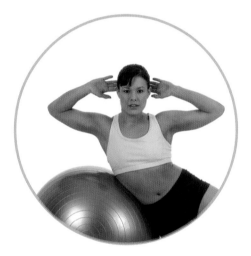

Hints

Control the movement through your midsection. Move slowly, trying to avoid jerky movements.

Keep your upper body upright, and do not allow your shoulders to fall forward or your elbows to come together.

ALTERNATING SUPERMAN

1 Lie facedown with the ball under your abdomen and both hands and feet touching the floor.

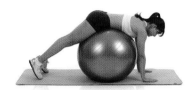

2 Raise one arm and the opposite leg off the floor, keeping them straight.

Lower your arm and leg back to the starting position.

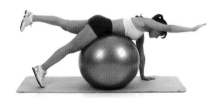

3 Repeat with your other arm and opposite leg.

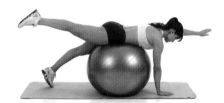

Hints

Keep the ball under your abdomen to maintain balance.

Raise your arm and leg in line with your hips and shoulders.

You should feel as if you are stretching out and lengthening your spine.

Exercise 8
CHAIR DIP

1 With the ball in front of you, position your hands on a chair, keeping your arms straight. Then place your feet on the ball with your legs straight.

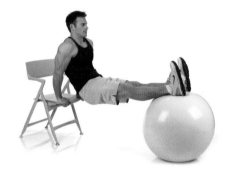

2 Lower your body toward the floor, bending at the elbows, dipping until your elbows are at shoulder level.

Push against the chair to return to the starting position where your arms are straight again.

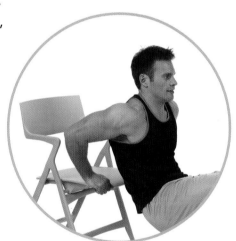

Hints

Start by sitting on the chair with your feet on the ball. Slowly push the ball out with your feet and position your hands on the edge of the chair. Be sure to use a sturdy chair that will support your weight.

Keep your head up, and look straight ahead to maintain a neutral back position. Deepen the dip when you feel comfortable with the exercise.

Exercise 9
SEATED TRUNK ROTATIONS

1 Sit upright on the ball with your hands on your hips.

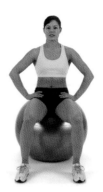

2 Rotate your midsection, making a big circle while still seated.

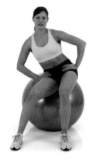

3 Repeat the movement in the opposite direction.

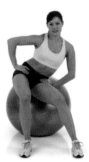

Hints

Keep contracting your core muscles throughout the movement.

Do not round your lower back as you complete the full range of motion.

Start with your feet shoulder-width apart. To increase the challenge to your stability, move your feet closer together.

Exercise 10
KNEELING BACK EXTENSION

1 Kneeling on the mat, place your chest on the ball and place your hands at the sides of your head.

Let your head and shoulders drape over the ball.

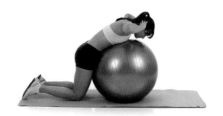

2 Lift your chest up off the ball, extending your back until your upper body is straight.

Keep your hands at the sides of your head, and return to the starting position.

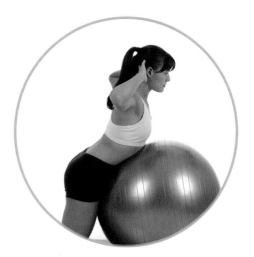

Hints

Lift only your head and shoulders, not your whole upper body.

Your upper body should be straight at the top of the movement.

Do not overarch your lower back.

WORKOUT 2

Exercise 1
SIDE LUNGE

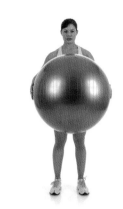

1 Stand with your feet hip-width apart, holding the ball at waist height.

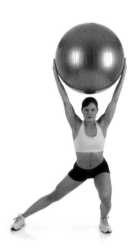

2 Step laterally to one side, lowering your body to a half-squat position, and raise the ball overhead with your arms fully extended.

Push off the outside foot to return to your starting position, and lower the ball to waist height.

Repeat the exercise with the other leg.

Hints

Always maintain a neutral back position. Do not round your lower back or overarch it.

Keep your head up, looking straight ahead, and your shoulders back. This will help prevent you from rounding your upper back.

Place your weight over the leg you step out with and push off this leg to return to the middle position. Keep the other leg straight.

Exercise 2
CRUNCH

1 Lie flat on your back on the mat, knees bent, with your heels on top of the ball.

Place your hands at the sides of your head.

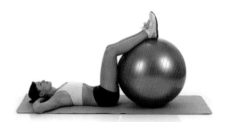

2 Lift your head and shoulders off the mat while contracting your abdominals.

Slowly roll your head and shoulders back to the mat, returning to the starting position.

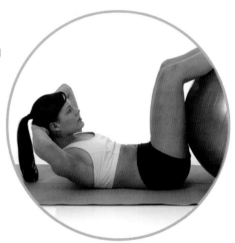

Hints
Make an effort to control the movement through your midsection, and avoid jerky movements.

Don't use your hands to pull up your head and neck.

Raise only your head and shoulders, not your whole back.

Exercise 3
SIDE ROTATION

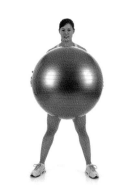

1 Stand upright, holding the ball at waist height.

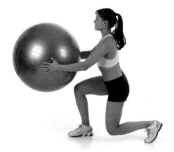

2 Rotate to one side, bending your hips and knees and lowering your body toward the floor. Switch sides, holding the ball at waist height throughout.

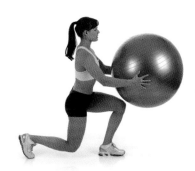

3 Repeat the movement in the opposite direction.

Hints

Keep your head up and look straight ahead throughout the movement. Do not look down at the floor or your feet.

Make sure to move your hips and feet as you move from side to side.

Keep the ball at waist height throughout.

Exercise 4
WALL PUSH-UP

1 Stand with your feet hip-width apart, facing a wall, holding the ball against the wall at chest height. Position your hands on the ball with your elbows bent and your chest nearly touching the ball.

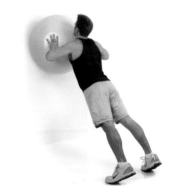

2 Push your body up and away from the ball until your arms are fully extended.

Slowly lower your body back to the starting position.

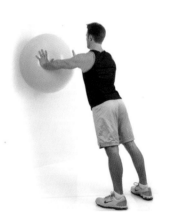

Hints

Keep your back straight by contracting your core muscles. Do not round your lower back.

Move all the way up and all the way down, until your chest is nearly touching the ball.

OVERHEAD DEADLIFT

1 Start in a squat position with your feet flat on the floor, head up, and your back in a neutral position.

Hold the ball on the floor in front of you.

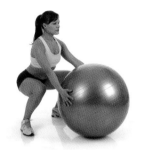

2 Stand up and lift the ball overhead with your arms fully extended.

Lower yourself back down so the ball is again on the floor in front of you.

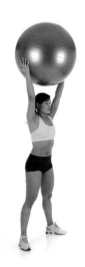

Hints

Your back position is very important in squatting exercises. Always maintain a neutral position.

Do not round your lower back or overarch it.

Keep your head up, looking straight ahead with your shoulders pulled back. This will help prevent rounding your upper back.

Exercise 6
ELBOW BRIDGE

1 Place your forearms on the ball and extend your legs with both feet on the floor.

The ball should be directly under your chest, and your body should be straight.

Hold this position for 20 seconds, then lower your body to lie on the ball.

Repeat in accordance with your chosen intensity level.

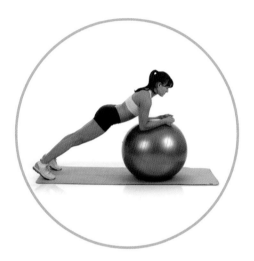

Hints

Start in a kneeling position with your elbows on the ball. Raise your hips and hold your torso in this position throughout the exercise.

Keep your forearms on top of the ball.

Start with your feet hip-width apart.

Exercise 7
LEG RAISE

1 Lie with your back on the mat, with the ball between your feet and your legs straight.

Place your hands by your sides.

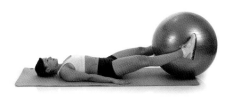

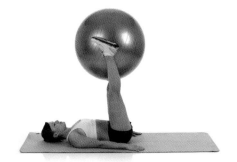

2 Raise your legs, keeping them straight, and lift the ball into position over your midsection.

Lower the ball, extending your hips to return to the starting position.

Hints

Keep your head, back, and shoulders on the mat.

Keep your legs straight.

Use your hands to help stabilize yourself, pushing them into the floor when lifting your hips.

Exercise 8
BALL LEG CURL

1 Lie with your back on the mat and your heels on the ball, with your legs extended. Raise your hips off the mat by contracting your abdominals. Place your hands by your sides.

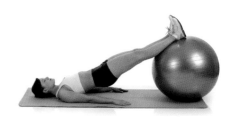

2 Pull the ball toward your buttocks, bending your knees.

Roll the ball from your heels to the bottom of your feet.

Extend your legs, returning the ball to the starting position with your heels back on the ball.

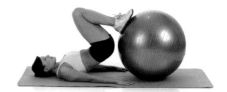

Hints
Keep your core and abdominal muscles contracted to maintain a neutral spine throughout the exercise.

Use your hands to help stabilize yourself, pushing them into the floor when drawing your knees in.

Exercise 9
DIP

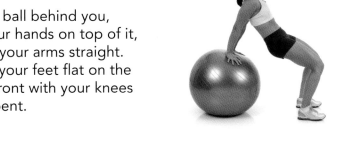

1 With the ball behind you, place your hands on top of it, keeping your arms straight. Position your feet flat on the floor in front with your knees slightly bent.

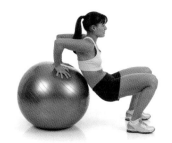

2 Lower your body toward the floor by bending your elbows and dipping down until your lower back touches the ball.

Push up against the ball until your arms are straight again, in the starting position.

Hints

You can position the ball against a wall to steady it.

Do not sit on the ball in the down position; barely touch the ball with your lower back.

Keep your feet flat on the floor throughout the exercise.

To increase the difficulty, straighten your legs and place your heels on the floor.

Keep your head up and look straight ahead.

Exercise 10
REVERSE BRIDGE

1 Lie with your back on the mat and your heels on top of the ball.

Place your hands by your sides on the mat.

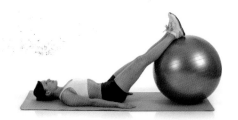

2 Lift your hips off the mat by contracting your core and abdominal muscles, and hold this position for 10 seconds.

Lower your body back to the mat, returning to the starting position.

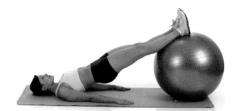

Hints

Keep your core and abdominal muscles contracted and maintain a neutral spine throughout the movement.

Use your hands to help stabilize yourself by pushing them into floor when raising your hips.

Only your head, upper back, and shoulders should touch the mat at the top position.

WORKOUT 3

Exercise 1
STEP UP

1 Start with your arms fully extended overhead, holding the ball in your hands.

Place one foot on a chair and the other foot flat on the floor.

Lean forward, shifting your body weight onto the foot on the chair.

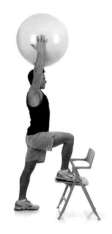

2 Push down on the foot on the chair, and using your core muscles, step up.

Keep the ball overhead with your arms fully extended. Finish your reps and repeat on the other side.

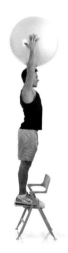

Hints
Keep your head up and look straight ahead to maintain a neutral spine.

Put your weight on the foot on the chair, not on the back foot.

Try not to push off using the back foot. Use the top leg to do the work.

Exercise 2
PUSH-UP

1 Lie facedown and place your hands on the mat directly under your shoulders and position your feet on the ball.

Your chest should nearly touch the mat with your body straight.

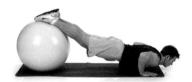

2 Push up and away from the mat, extending your arms fully.

Lower your body down to the mat until your chest is again nearly touching it.

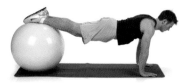

Hints

Start by lying on your stomach on the ball and walking your hands out while rolling the ball down your legs to your feet.

Go all the way down until your chest is nearly touching the mat, and then push back up, extending your arms fully.

Look down at the floor to maintain a neutral spine. Do not move your head.

Exercise 3
REVERSE CRUNCH

1 Lie back on the mat. Position the ball on the mat between your feet with your knees bent.

Place your hands at your sides.

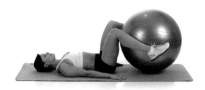

2 Raise your hips and lower back off the mat, bringing your knees to your chest, and lifting the ball up.

Return to the starting position with the ball on the mat.

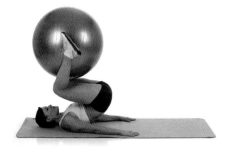

Hints

Keep your upper back and shoulders on the mat.

Do not move your legs. Keep your knees bent at the same angle throughout the exercise.

Complete the full range of motion, returning the ball to the mat every time.

Exercise 4
UNI OVERHEAD DEADLIFT

1 Squat in front of the ball with your feet flat on the floor, your head up, and your back in a neutral position.

Raise one foot off the floor and grasp the ball with your hands in front of you.

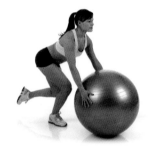

2 Stand up and lift the ball overhead with your arms fully extended, keeping one foot off the floor.

Squat down on one leg, returning to the starting position, and setting the ball on the floor.

Repeat with your other leg.

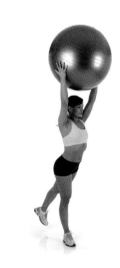

Hints
Keep your abdominal and core muscles activated during the exercise. Do not round your lower back.

Your standing leg should remain straight throughout the exercise. A slight bend at the knee may help people with flexibility limitations.

Exercise 5
CHAIR DIP

1 With the ball in front of you, position your hands on a chair, keeping your arms straight. Then place your feet on the ball with your legs straight.

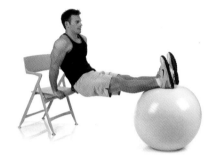

2 Lower your body toward the floor, bending at the elbows, dipping until your elbows are at shoulder level.

Push against the chair to return to the starting position, where your arms are straight again.

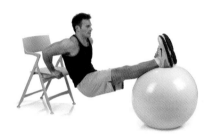

Hints

Start by sitting on the chair with your feet on the ball. Slowly push the ball out with your feet and position your hands on the edge of the chair. Be sure to use a sturdy chair that will support your weight.

Keep your head up, and look straight ahead to maintain a neutral back position.

Deepen the dip when you feel comfortable with the exercise.

WORKOUT 3

SIDE BRIDGE

1 Lean to one side with your forearm on the ball and your legs stretched out.

Place your other arm on your side.

Raise your hips off the ball.

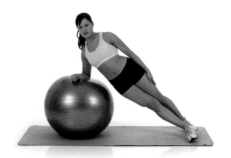

2 Hold this position for 20 seconds, then lower your hips back down to the ball.

Repeat to complete your reps, then switch sides.

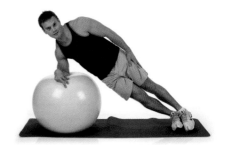

Hints

Lie with your side on the ball. Raise your hips off the ball and hold this position.

Do not let your hips sag or dip. This will require you to contract the abdominal and core muscles.

Keep your upper body aligned with your hips. Do not allow your shoulders to fall forward.

Look straight ahead to maintain a neutral spine.

Exercise 7
OBLIQUE BACK EXTENSION

1 Lie facedown with your chest on the ball with your hands at the sides of your head and your legs extended.

Let your head and shoulders drape over the ball.

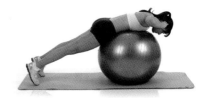

2 Lift your chest up off the ball, extending through your back, and rotate your upper body to one side.

Keep your hands at the sides of your head, and return to the starting position with your chest on the ball.

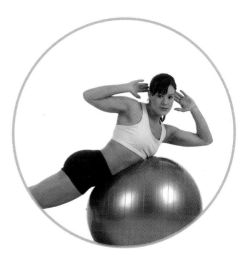

Hints
Lift just your head and shoulders, not your whole upper body.

Keep your shoulders aligned. Do not allow your upper body to fall forward.

Do not overarch your lower back.

Push your toes into the floor to help stabilize you and prevent slipping.

Exercise 8
ROLL OUT

1 Kneel on the mat with your forearms on the ball, your elbows bent, and your chest nearly touching the ball.

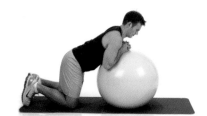

2 Push the ball forward, extending your arms and keeping your upper body rigid.

Pull the ball back, drawing your elbows in until you reach the starting position.

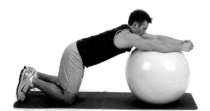

Hints

Maintain a neutral spine by looking down and not moving your head.

Control the movement through your midsection, and avoid jerky movements. This requires you to keep your abdominal and core muscles contracted throughout the exercise.

Exercise 9
ALTERNATING SUPERMAN

1 Lie facedown with the ball under your abdomen and both hands and feet touching the floor.

2 Raise one arm and the opposite leg off the floor, keeping them straight.

Lower your arm and leg back to the starting position.

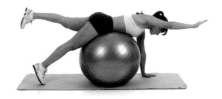

3 Repeat with your other arm and opposite leg.

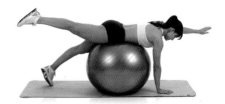

Hints

Keep the ball under your abdomen to maintain balance.

Raise your arm and leg in line with your hips and shoulders.

You should feel as if you are stretching out and lengthening your spine.

Exercise 10
OBLIQUE CRUNCH

1 Lie with your side on the ball with both legs extended and both feet on the mat. Place your hands at the sides of your head.

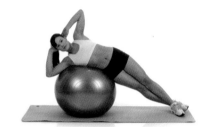

2 Raise your upper body up and off the ball, bringing your outside elbow down to your side.

Lower your body, returning to the starting position, lying over the ball.

Complete your reps and repeat on the other side.

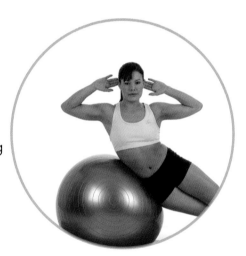

Hints

Control the movement through your midsection. Move slowly, trying to avoid jerky movements.

Keep your upper body upright, and do not allow your shoulders to fall forward or your elbows to come together.

Exercise 1
SPLIT SQUAT

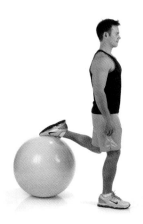

1 Stand with the ball on the floor behind you.

Place one foot on top of the ball and the other positioned out in front on the floor.

Place your bodyweight on the leg out in front.

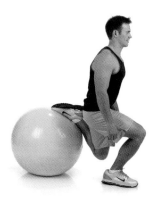

2 Lower your body until your back shin touches the ball.

Keep your back in a neutral position.

Push through the front foot to return to the starting position.

Complete your reps and repeat on the other side.

Hints

The position of your back is very important in performing squatting exercises. Always maintain a neutral spinal position. Do not round your lower back or overarch it.

Keep your head up and look straight ahead to maintain a neutral spine.

Put your body weight on the foot out in front, not on the back foot.

Exercise 2
TWISTING CRUNCH

1 Lie on your back over the ball and center the ball in your mid-back.

Keep your head and neck off the ball and your feet flat on the floor.

Place your hands at the sides of your head.

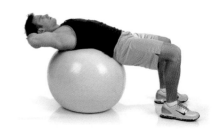

2 Lift your head and shoulders up and away from the ball and twist to one side, contracting your abdominals and twisting through your midsection.

Twist back to the center and roll your upper body back over the ball, returning to the starting position.

Complete your reps and repeat on the other side.

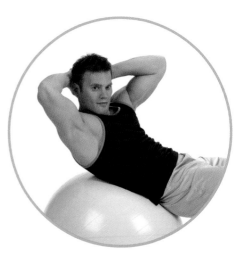

Hints

Control the movement through your midsection, and avoid jerky movements.

Do not use your hands to pull your head and neck up.

Lift only your head and shoulders, not your whole back.

Start with your feet shoulder-width apart. To make it more challenging, bring your feet closer together.

Exercise 3
PUSH-UP

1 Start with your hands on the ball directly under your shoulders and your legs extended with your feet hip-width apart on the floor.

Your chest should be nearly touching the ball, and your body should be fully extended.

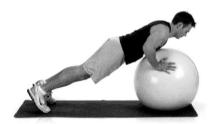

2 Push up away from the ball, until your arms are fully extended.

Lower your body down to the ball, returning to the starting position. Again, your chest should nearly touch the ball.

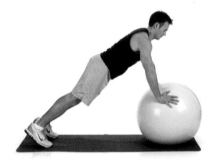

Hints

Go all the way down until your chest is nearly touching the ball, and then push back up, extending your arms fully.

Look down at the floor to maintain a neutral spine. Do not move your head.

Exercise 4
UNI STIFF LEG DEADLIFT

1 Stand upright with your arms extended in front of your chest, holding the ball.

Raise one foot off the floor.

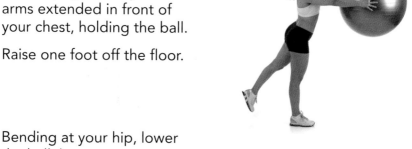

2 Bending at your hip, lower the ball, keeping your arms and the standing leg straight.

Lower to the point where your shoulders are hip level and your lifted leg is parallel to the floor, then return to the starting position.

Repeat and switch legs.

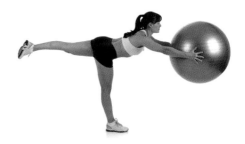

Hints

Keep your abdominal and core muscles activated during the exercise. Do not round your lower back.

Your standing leg should remain straight throughout the exercise. A slight bend at the knee may help people with flexibility limitations.

Exercice 5
ARM TO LEG TRANSFER

1 Lie on your back on the mat with your legs straight and slightly off the floor, your arms overhead, and hold the ball in your hands.

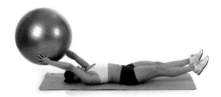

2 Simultaneously raise your arms and legs, keeping them straight to bring the ball over your midsection. Transfer the ball from your hands to between your feet.

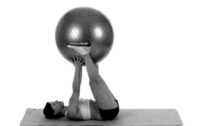

3 Lower both your arms and legs, returning to the starting position, with the ball now between your feet.

Reverse the movement.

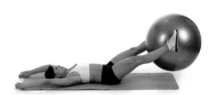

Hints
Keep your arms and legs straight throughout the exercise.

If you like, set your feet on the mat at the end of each repetition. To increase the difficulty, keep your feet off the mat at all times.

Exercise 6
DIP

1 With the ball behind you, place your hands on top of it, keeping your arms straight. Position your feet flat on the floor in front with your knees slightly bent.

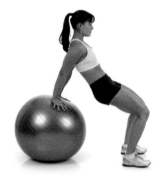

2 Lower your body toward the floor by bending your elbows and dipping down until your lower back touches the ball.

Push up against the ball until your arms are straight again, in the starting position.

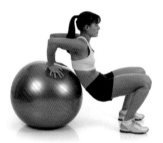

Hints

You can position the ball against a wall to steady it.

Do not sit on the ball in the down position; barely touch the ball with your lower back.

Keep your head up and look straight ahead.

Keep your feet flat on the floor throughout the exercise.

To increase the difficulty, straighten your legs and place your heels on the floor.

Exercise 7
LOWER BODY TWIST

1 Lie with your back on the mat, with your knees bent and the ball between your knees, off the floor.

Place your hands at your sides.

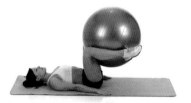

2 Rotate your lower body to one side until that knee touches the floor, still holding the ball between your knees.

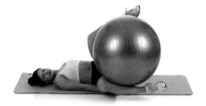

3 Rotate 180 degrees to the other side, and repeat, touching the floor with your other knee.

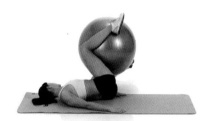

Hints
Keep your shoulders and upper back on the mat throughout the exercise.

Twist through your midsection, using your abdominal muscles to move yourself.

Exercise 8
UNI BALL CURL

1 Lie with your back on the mat and your heels on the ball, with your legs extended.

Raise your hips by contracting your abdominals.

Place your hands by your sides, and hold this position. Lift one foot off the ball.

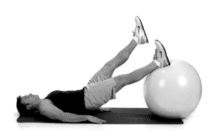

2 Pull the ball toward your buttocks, with the leg on the ball, bending your knee. Keep your other leg straight.

Roll the ball from your heel to the bottom of your foot. Extend your leg, returning the ball to the starting position with one heel on the ball.

Complete your reps and repeat with the other leg.

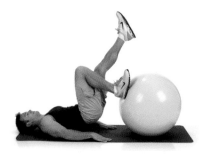

Hints

Keep your core and abdominal muscles contracted to maintain a neutral spine throughout the exercise.

Use your hands to help stabilize yourself, pushing them into the floor when drawing your knee in.

Exercise 9
BRIDGE

1 Place your hands on the ball with your arms and legs extended and your feet on the floor hip-width apart.

The ball should be directly under your chest. Hold your body straight.

Hold this position for 20 seconds, then lower your body to lie on the ball.

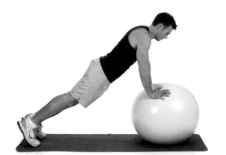

Hints

Keep your core and abdominal muscles contracted and maintain a neutral spine throughout the movement.

Exercise 10
UNI REVERSE BRIDGE

1 Lie on your back on the mat with your heels on the ball and legs extended.

Place your hands by your sides, and raise one foot off the ball.

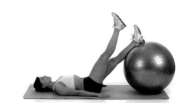

2 Raise your hips off the mat, contracting your abdominals, and hold this position.

Lower your hips back to the mat, returning to the starting position, keeping one leg off the ball.

Complete your reps and repeat with the other leg.

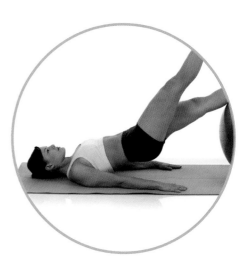

Hints

Keep your core and abdominal muscles contracted to maintain a neutral spinal position throughout the exercise.

Use your hands to help stabilize yourself. Push them into the floor while raising your hips.

Only your head, upper back, and shoulders should contact the mat at the top position.

Stretch 1
HAMSTRINGS 1

Stand with one heel on the ball positioned in front of you.

Hold your arms out in front of you, and gently lean forward at the waist, stretching your hands toward your foot.

INTENSITY

Hold for 10 seconds

Repeat 3 times with each leg

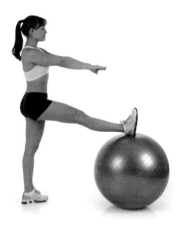
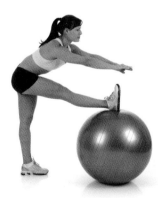

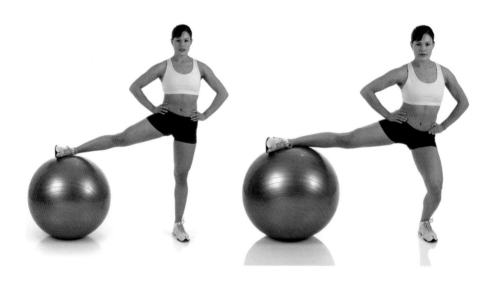

STRETCHING

Stretch 2
ADDUCTORS

Stand with the inside ankle
of one leg on the ball.

Slowly lower your body into
a half squat, stretching the
inside of the leg on the ball.

INTENSITY

Hold for 10 seconds

Repeat 3 times with
each leg

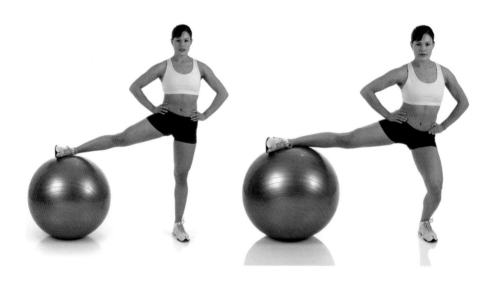

Stretch 3
QUADRICEPS

Lie facedown over the ball, positioning it in your midsection. Start with both hands and feet on the floor.

Raise one leg, bending at the knee, and hold the ankle with your hand.

Pull your foot toward your buttocks.

INTENSITY

Hold for 10 seconds

Repeat 3 times with each leg

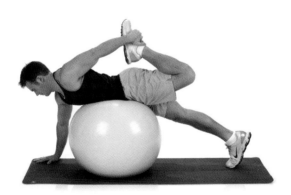

STRETCHING

Stretch 4
BACK 1

Lie facedown with the ball centered under your midsection.

Place your hands and feet on the floor, and let your head and shoulders fall forward over the ball.

Lengthen your spine as you stretch over the ball.

INTENSITY

Hold for 10 seconds

Repeat 3 times

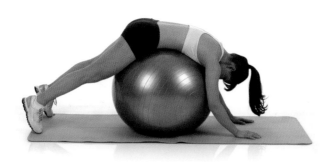

BACK 2

Lie facedown over the ball, centering your midsection, with your feet and hands on the floor. Raise one arm and rotate at your waist until your arm is overhead and directly in line with the hand on the floor. Look up at the hand overhead.

INTENSITY

Hold for 10 seconds

Repeat 3 times on each side

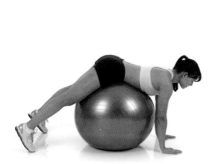 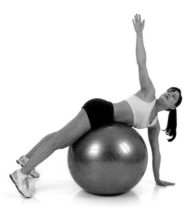

STRETCHING

Stretch 6
TRICEPS

Sit upright on the ball with
one arm, bent at the elbow,
behind your head.

Place the other hand on
that elbow, and slowly pull
it across to the middle of
your back.

INTENSITY

Hold for 10 seconds

Repeat 3 times with
each arm

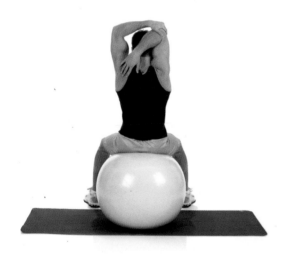

CHEST

Lie with your back on the ball and your arms stretched overhead.

Roll back so the ball rests in your mid-back with your head, shoulders, and arms hanging over it. Lower your hands toward the floor and lengthen your spine.

INTENSITY

Hold for 10 seconds

Repeat 3 times

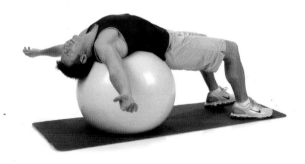

STRETCHING

Stretch 8
HAMSTRINGS 2

Lie with your back on the mat. Place one leg on the ball with your knee bent.

Keep the other leg straight, and clasp your hands behind your calf.

Slowly pull the straight leg toward your head.

INTENSITY

Hold for 10 seconds

Repeat 3 times with each leg

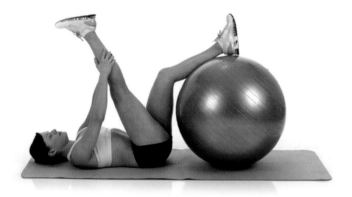

Stretch 9
GLUTES

Lie with your back on the mat. Place one leg on the ball with your knee bent.

Place the other ankle across that knee. Gently push the outside knee away from you.

INTENSITY

Hold for 10 seconds

Repeat 3 times with each leg

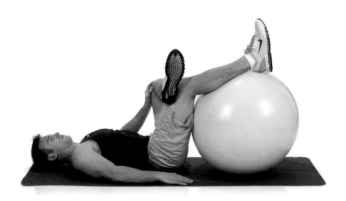

STRETCHING

Stretch 10
ABDUCTOR

Lie on your side with your lower leg on the ball, and the other leg behind it.

Push down on the ball with your leg, and raise your upper body off the mat.

INTENSITY

Hold for 10 seconds

Repeat 3 times with each leg

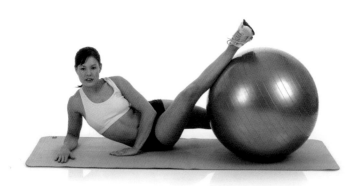

INDEX

Abdominals
    Arm to Leg Transfer, 47
    Ball Crunch, 15
    Crunch, 24
    Kneeling Oblique Crunch, 18
    Leg Raise, 29
    Lower Body Twist, 49
    Oblique Crunch, 42
    Reverse Bridge, 32
    Reverse Crunch, 35
    Seated Trunk Rotations, 21
    Side Bridge, 38
    Side Rotation, 25
    Twisting Crunch, 44
    Uni Reverse Bridge, 52

Alternating Superman, 19, 41

Arm to Leg Transfer, 47

Arms
    Chair Dip, 20, 37
    Dip, 31, 48

Back
    Alternating Superman, 19, 41
    Ball Leg Curl, 30
    Bridge, 51
    Elbow Bridge, 28
    Kneeling Back Extension, 22
    Oblique Back Extension, 39

Ball Crunch, 15

Ball Leg Curl, 30

Ball sizes, 8

Benefits, of Swiss ball, 4–5

Book, organization of, 8–9

Bridge, 51

Chair Dip, 20, 37

Chest
    Push-Up, 34, 45
    Wall Push-Up, 14, 26

Cool down, 7, 12

Coordination, improving, 4–5

Core
    defined, 5
    posture and, 6
    Swiss ball and, 5

Crunch, 24

Dip, 31, 48

Doctor, consulting, 7

Elbow Bridge, 28

Equipment, 8

Exercises
    getting started, 10
    intensity tracks, 8–9
    total health plan and, 9

Express track, 8

Intense track, 8

Intensity tracks, 8

Kneeling, on ball, 10

Kneeling Back Extension, 22

Kneeling Oblique Crunch, 18

Leg Raise, 29

Legs
    Lunge, 16
    Overhead Deadlift, 27
    Overhead Squat, 13
    Side Lunge, 23

Legs (con't)
    Split Squat, 43
    Step Up, 33
    Uni Ball Curl, 50
    Uni Overhead Deadlift, 36
    Uni Stiff Leg Deadlift, 46
Lower Body Twist, 49
Lunge, 16
Lying on ball, 10
Muscle synergy, 5
Oblique Back Extension, 39
Oblique Crunch, 42
Organization of book, 8–9
Overhead Deadlift, 27
Overhead Squat, 13
Proprioception, 4–5
Push-Up, 34, 45
Reverse Bridge, 32
Reverse Crunch, 35
Roll Out, 17, 40
Safety precautions, 7–8
Seated Trunk Rotations, 21
Side Bridge, 38
Side Lunge, 23
Side Rotation, 25
Sitting on ball, 10
Sizes, of ball, 8
Split Squat, 43

Starting exercise program, 10
Step Up, 33
Stretches
    Abductor, 62
    Adductors, 54
    Back 1, 56
    Back 2, 57
    Chest, 59
    Glutes, 61
    Hamstrings 1, 53
    Hamstrings 2, 60
    Quadriceps, 55
    Triceps, 58
Swiss ball
    back and, 6
    benefits of, 4–5
    size guidelines, 8
Twisting Crunch, 44
Uni Ball Curl, 50
Uni Overhead Deadlift, 36
Uni Reverse Bridge, 52
Uni Stiff Leg Deadlift, 46
Variety, 5
Wall Push-Up, 14, 26
Warm-up, 12
Workout 1, 13–22
Workout 2, 23–32
Workout 3, 33–42
Workout 4, 43–52